Clinical Standards Advisory Group:

Schizophrenia. Volume 2

Protocol for Assessing Services for People with Severe Mental Illness

Report of a CSAG Committee on Schizophrenia: Volume 2

John Wing, Susannah Rix, Roy Curtis
College Research Unit, 11 Grosvenor Crescent, London, SW1X 7EE.

July 1995

London HMSO

© Crown Copyright 1995

Applications for reproduction should be made to HMSO's Copyright Unit

ISBN 0 11 321 922 9

Other titles in this series of CSAG reports are available from HMSO Books and include:

Access to and Availability of Specialist Services
0 11 321 596 7

Coronary Artery Bypass Grafting and Coronary Angioplasty: access to and availability of specialist services
0 11 321 597 5

Childhood Leukaemia: access to and availability of specialist services
0 11 321 598 3

Neonatal Intensive Care: access to and availability of specialist services
0 11 321 599 1

Cystic Fibrosis: access and availabilty to specialist services
0 11 321 600 9

Standards of Clinical Care for People with Diabetes
0 11 321 819 2

Back Pain
0 11 321 887 7

Epidemiology Review: the Epidemiology and Cost of Back Pain
0 11 321 889 3

Urgent and Emergency Admissions to Hospital
0 11 321 835 4

Dental General Anaesthesia
0 11 321 924 5

Women in Normal Labour
0 11 321 923 7

Schizophrenia Volume 1
0 11 321 929 6

ABOUT HMSO's STANDING ORDER SERVICE

The Standing Order service, open to all HMSO account holders★, allows customers to receive automatically the publications they require in a specified subject area, thereby saving them the time, trouble and expense of placing individual orders.

Customers may choose from over 4,000 classifications arranged in more than 250 sub groups under 30 major subject areas. These classifications enable customers to choose from a wide range of subjects those publications which are of special interest to them. This is a particularly valuable service for the specialist library or research body. All publications will be despatched to arrive immediately after publication date. A special leaflet describing the service in detail may be obtained on request.

Write to Standing Order Service, HMSO Books, PO Box 276, LONDON SW8 5DT quoting classification reference 14.01.027 to order future titles in this series.

★Details of requirements to open an account can be obtained from HMSO Books, PO Box 276, London SW8 5DT.

Contents

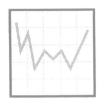

Preface to Volume 2

This is the second of the two volumes of CSAG's report on Schizophrenia. Volume 1 is the main report; Volume 2 is a revision of the protocol used by CSAG in 1994.

CSAG

The Clinical Standards Advisory Group (CSAG) was established in April 1991, under Section 62 of the National Health Service (NHS) and Community Care Act 1990, as an independent source of expert advice to the UK Health Ministers and to the NHS on standards of clinical care for, and access to and availability of services to, NHS patients. Remits are set by the UK Health Ministers in discussion with the Group. The Group's members are nominated by the medical, nursing and dental Royal Colleges and their Faculties, and include the Chairmen of the Standing Medical, Nursing and Midwifery, and Dental Advisory Committees. Its investigations are carried out by members and co-opted experts, supported by research units under contract – in this case the Royal College of Psychiatrists' Research Unit. Financial support is provided by the UK Health Departments, and the secretariat is based in the Department of Health, Room 409, Wellington House, 133/155 Waterloo Road, London, SE1 8UG.

Volume 1

Volume 1 was published by HMSO in July 1995, ISBN 011 321 929 6, price £15. It reports on the creation of a protocol of guidelines on services for people with schizophrenia and other severe mental illnesses, and its use in eleven UK health districts.

Volume 2

Volume 2 forms part of CSAG's report but is also available separately, without charge from:

Health Publications Unit
Heywood Stores
Manchester Road
Heywood
Lancashire OL10 2BZ

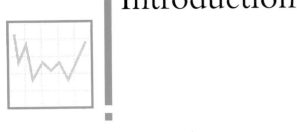

Introduction

The first volume of this report described the creation of a protocol of guidelines on services for people with schizophrenia and other severe mental illnesses, and its use in eleven UK health districts. One of the conclusions reached in Volume 1 was that the experiences of members of the visiting teams and of CSAG's Schizophrenia committee should be drawn upon to draft an improved version of the protocol. Appendix 3 of Volume 1 contained a list of guidelines that team members suggested should be considered in any revision. Some of the original consultants were also asked to comment.

A revised draft was produced incorporating these suggestions and circulated to all who had been involved with the project, either directly or indirectly, with a request for detailed annotations and an invitation to attend a one-day workshop at which the latest draft would be fully discussed. This took place on 10 April 1995 and was very successful. The final version 2 of the protocol is therefore based on a substantial programme of consultation and practical experience.

Changes from version 1

The main change is that the 'key point' system used to provide an overview of the results of the field trials has become part of the new structure. There are now 9 Purchaser Sections in Part 1 and 17 Provider Sections in Part 2, including one on morale. Each section has one general quality rating so that an overall profile of performance is immediately accessible. Account is taken of the fact that each 'district' can contain more than one hospital ward, several community teams, and many versions of community facilities. There are fewer numbered items within sections but prompts for most items are now conveniently listed on the page opposite the section ratings. The whole schedule is now simpler to administer while covering more ground.

There are still gaps. In particular, the sections dealing with primary care/GPFH, Social Services, and users and carers, none of which was in the original remit, could be developed further. Standards for treatments such as medication, cognitive therapy, family support, etc, are not included, since they are more suited to individual clinical audit and are difficult to assess during a brief visit to a district.

Users are reminded that the Protocol Version 2 is intended to be used as part of the audit cycle. Each cross-section provides a profile of good and not-so-good practice, which should suggest appropriate action, the outcome of which is further audited.

Definition of 'severe mental illness'

In its document on interagency collaboration, the Department has recommended including schizophrenia and severe affective disorder (subchapters F2 and F3 of ICD-10) associated with florid current symptoms, recurrent crises, or serious current or long-term disability. These make up the large proportion of problems likely to be considered while using the protocol. Other disorders (e.g. from F4, neurotic, stress-related and somatoform disorders or F5, behavioural syndromes) may also fit the description if the crisis or disability caused is severe, but numbers are much smaller. The protocol is not intended for use with services primarily focused on dementia, personality disorders, learning or developmental disorders, or those of childhood or adolescence.

The rating scales

The scales are listed both at the front of Version 2 of the Protocol and on a fold out section in the back. Ratings are entered opposite the relevant guideline on the right-hand page.
Scale A is used to assess how far services have taken action to ensure that individual guidelines have been met.
Scale B is for rating overall quality. A rating of 4 would usually mean one or more examples of very good practice, which should be recorded on the left-hand page. Similarly, examples of poor practice should be noted for action. The term 'average' is no longer used because of the confusion caused by its use in two different ways, absolute and statistical. Each rating of quality on scale B is made purely as a judgement of how far the guidelines in the Section under review are met by the particular service under scrutiny. Scores can later be derived that can be used for comparative purposes.
Scale C measures only the accessibility of services. It is not possible to cover the quality or suitability of the service in the same rating. A and B do that.
Scale D provides a means of identifying the organisation responsible for supplying or funding a service.
The PAG scale is an optional means of checking the quality of residential accommodation against a comprehensive checklist of criteria. It is particularly useful as an aid to making an overall judgement when several different examples of housing are under scrutiny,
while keeping a record of any variation in quality.

The volumes, activities and population indicators collected will be decided locally.

Uses

Volume 1 of the report demonstrates some of the ways in which scores can be used. It is legitimate to make statistical comparisons so long as key variables such as background socio-economic factors, availability of resources, and recent organisational stability are taken into account. Application of the principles of the audit cycle will allow a wide variety of local uses intended to locate and rectify specific problems. This flexibility will be important as the scope of the commissioning process and the populations covered develops further. Finally it should be borne in mind that version 2 has received only a first trial, on the basis of which is has been improved. It will benefit from further modification in the light of experience.

Part 1: Purchasing Mental Health Services

		Scale B
1.1:	Mental Health Needs Assessment	0 1 2 3 4
1.2:	Purchasing Strategy	0 1 2 3 4
1.3:	Commissioning & the Interaction Between Purchasers & Providers	0 1 2 3 4
1.4:	The Service Specification & Contract(s) for Mental Health Services	0 1 2 3 4
1.5:	Contract Monitoring & the Requirements for Information	0 1 2 3 4
1.6:	Implementation, Quality & Audit Procedures	0 1 2 3 4
1.7:	Interactions with other Purchasers (GPFH & LASS)	0 1 2 3 4
1.8:	General Practitioner Fundholding	0 1 2 3 4
1.9:	Local Authority Social Services	0 1 2 3 4

Scale A - Action to meet guideline

0	No action yet taken, few plans	3	Guideline is substantially met
1	Plans, little action	4	Guideline is fully met or exceeded
2	Guideline is partially met	9	Not known, or not applicable

Section 1.1 Assessment includes:

1.1.1   Use is made of national information/indicators

Use is made of local information/indicators

Specifically:

- indices of poverty, unemployment, deprivation
- social isolation, marital status, migration
- ethnicity
- SMR, age and sex structure
- other sociodemographic variables
- geographical factors, service access, housing

1.1.2   National guidelines

Health of the Nation targets: improved functioning

Decreased rates of suicide

Patients' Charter

1.1.3   More than extrapolation from national data

More than extrapolation from local needs assessment in areas other than mental health

Evidence of a systematic approach, including small area/practice-based needs assessment

Evidence of active involvement of other stakeholders

1.1.4   See Health Promotion Strategy/Annual Report etc.

Section 1.1: Mental Health Needs Assessment

1.1.1   Mental health needs assessment is based on population indicators for severe mental illness   **A 0 1 2 3 4**

1.1.2   Needs assessment includes consideration of national guidelines and targets   **A 0 1 2 3 4**

1.1.3   There is a systematic approach towards mental health needs assessment   **A 0 1 2 3 4**

1.1.4   Health promotion activities include: **A 0 1 2 3 4**
- specific initiatives aimed at those with SMI
- specific reference to those with SMI in general health promotion activities

SUMMARY RATING FOR SECTION 1.1:	**Scale B:**	**0**	**1**	**2**	**3**	**4**

Section 1.2 Assessment includes:

1.2 Purchasers have a clear written strategy for commissioning high quality services. The strategy documentation demonstrates expertise in both mental health and strategy formulation.

1.2.2 Providers
Other purchasers,
Others involved in the development and review of the purchasing strategy

1.2.3 Explicit justification is provided if strategy differs

1.2.4 There are specific strategies for both major and minor mental health problems

1.2.5 Shared recognition of severe mental illness
Shared understanding of District needs
Regular consultations with stakeholders
Shared budgets/budget planning
Clear and agreed allocation of responsibilities

1.2.6

	Informed	Consulted	Involved
Provider, managers, clinicians			
Social Services			
GPs/FHSA			
GPFHs			
Non-statutory providers			
User/carer			
L.A. housing/L.A. employment			

Section 1.2: Purchasing Strategy

1.2.1   A definition of severe mental illness is explicit in the purchasing strategy **A   0   1   2   3   4**

1.2.2   The definition of severe mental illness is shared with and **A   0   1   2   3   4**
         agreed by all relevant parties

1.2.3   The problems characteristic of severe mental illness are to be targeted **A   0   1   2   3   4**

1.2.4   There is reference to the full range of mental health problems **A   0   1   2   3   4**

1.2.5   The strategy informs the purchasing plan and contract negotiations **A   0   1   2   3   4**

1.2.6   The strategy provides a basis for collaboration with local providers and purchasers, and **A   0   1   2   3   4**
         shows evidence of the involvement of all parties in its development, monitoring and review

1.2.7   The strategy contains, or is supported by, a clear implementation **A   0   1   2   3   4**
         or development plan

SUMMARY RATING FOR SECTION 1.2:	Scale B:	0	1	2	3	4

Section 1.3 Assessment includes:

1.3.1   Context in which decisions for purchasing mental health services are made.

Team should record name and grade of person with lead responsibility for purchasing mental health services.

1.3.2   Differentiate from consultation on strategy (see 1.2.6)
- process of negotiation should include:
- contract monitoring
- development /review of service specification
- local users and carers
- relevant and representative direct care staff
- provider service managers
- general practitioners
- social services
- other local authority representatives (if not included in social services representation)

Section 1.3: Commissioning & the Interaction Between Purchasers & Providers

1.3.1   Purchasing decisions for mental health services are made in the context of experienced of mental health service needs and delivery   **A   0 1 2 3 4**

1.3.2   The process of contract negotiation involves the active participation of all relevant parties   **A   0 1 2 3 4**

1.3.3   The purchasing organisation is represented in these negotiations by senior officers, of whom at least one is a director (or equivalent)   **A   0 1 2 3 4**

SUMMARY RATING FOR SECTION 1.3:	Scale B:	0	1	2	3	4

Section 1.4 Assessment includes:

1.4.2   Standards may be either nationally or locally derived

Targets may be either nationally or locally derived

The documentation sets out:

- prioritisation for SMI
- acute and emergency care
- longer term secure care
- longer term residential care
- other sheltered accommodation
- rehabilitation and daytime activity
- information for patients and carers
- support for advocacy for users and carers
- details of specific standards and targets and methods of monitoring and reviewing these

Section 1.4: The Service Specification & Contract(s) for Mental Health Services

1.4.1   There is a separate service specification and specific contract(s) for mental health   **A   0   1   2   3   4**
         services, with a specified budget

1.4.2   Services for people with severe mental illness are specifically identified, and budgeted for,   **A   0   1   2   3   4**
         in the contract documentation, including information on costs, volumes, standards and targets.

SUMMARY RATING FOR SECTION 1.4:	**Scale B:**	**0**	**1**	**2**	**3**	**4**

Section 1.5 Assessment includes:

1.5.1   Avoid perverse incentives,

e.g.   • reference to open access to services is qualified (targeting must mean restricted access)
   • specific conditions are imposed if healthcare professionals skilled with SMI work in primary care settings
   • avoid premature discharge from care of patients judged unlikely to improve
   • avoid use of simple cost/volume formulae in community settings where intention is to prioritise SMI (thus reducing caseload volumes)

1.5.2   Information includes:
   • WHO: is involved in contract monitoring (on purchaser and provider sides)
   • WHEN: frequency of meetings
   • WHY: what is the declared purpose of contract monitoring; how is information and feedback used in revising the contract, developing the contract currency etc.
   • WHAT: what currency is used; what information is required for monitoring; what, if any, incentives/bonuses/sanctions are included

1.5.3   Patient bed days/out-patient activity/other activity indicators – specify
   CPA ' activity' (e.g. numbers, levels)
   Care protocols (e.g. CPA monitoring tool) – specify
   Outcome indicators (e.g. HoNOS) – specify
   Others   i) general – e.g. incident reporting
          ii) specific – e.g. to monitor specific local services or developments such as individual care packages, court diversion schemes etc.

Section 1.5: Contract Monitoring & the Requirements for Information

1.5.1   Perverse incentives are avoided in the commissioning process and contract data set   **A   0 1 2 3 4**

1.5.2   The contract documentation specifies arrangements for monitoring the agreed contract   **A   0 1 2 3 4**

1.5.3   The contract specifies a full range of relevant currencies   **A   0 1 2 3 4**

SUMMARY RATING FOR SECTION 1.5:	**Scale B:**	**0**	**1**	**2**	**3**	**4**

Section 1.6 Assessment includes:

1.6.1   Should include:
- CPA
- Care management
- Section 117
- Mental Health Act Code of Practice
- Supervision register
- Supervised discharge (when appropriate)
- Health of the Nation targets
- Patients Charter - relevant standards and targets

1.6.4   A senior person has responsibility for 'quality' issues (i.e. board level, or reporting to board level officer)

Regular clinical audit required

Regular medical audit required

Written records/reports of audit sessions available

Audit protocols are agreed - including specific protocols for SMI

Monitoring or other mechanisms in place to ensure that audit outcomes change practice

The purchaser has specific input to the choice of topics/areas for audit (e.g. an agreed percentage of time or number of topics is determined by the purchaser)

1.6.5   e.g. skilled family intervention, defined budgets for specific medications

1.6.6   Compare contracts from previous years

Ask for examples

Section 1.6: Implementation, Quality & Audit Procedures

1.6.1   The contract requires the implementation of all relevant statutory and policy directives   **A   0 1 2 3 4**

1.6.2   Annual targets are set, published and circulated widely   **A   0 1 2 3 4**

1.6.3   There is a quality assurance strategy for services for people with severe mental illness   **A   0 1 2 3 4**

1.6.4   Quality is ensured through explicit mechanisms   **A   0 1 2 3 4**

1.6.5   Specific treatments and interventions for people with severe mental illness are   **A   0 1 2 3 4**
identified; their availability and effectiveness is subject to monitoring and/or audit

1.6.6   There is clear evidence that the purchaser uses information derived from contract monitoring,   **A   0 1 2 3 4**
quality assurance and audit monitoring to inform and modify the contract or service specification

SUMMARY RATING FOR SECTION 1.6:	Scale B:	0	1	2	3	4

Section 1.7 Assessment includes:

1.7.2   Boundary issues – i.e. who is responsible for purchasing what and where

1.7.3   See relevant documents

Section 1.7: Interactions with other Purchasers (GPFH & LASS)

1.7.1   DHA purchaser has agreement of other purchasers on its strategy and prioritisation   **A 0 1 2 3 4**
of severe mental illness

1.7.2   DHA purchaser has agreed with other purchasers: **A 0 1 2 3 4**
- boundary issues
- procedures for resolving differences
- groundrules for ECRs
- budget levels, shared budgets, rules for virement

1.7.3   The priorities and targets within the DHAs strategic plan are consistent with those in   **A 0 1 2 3 4**
the Community Care Plan (q.v.) and with other documents with joint authorship

SUMMARY RATING FOR SECTION 1.7:	Scale B:	0	1	2	3	4

Section 1.8 Assessment includes:

1.8.1 Employing skilled mental health practitioners to work in the practice
Regular audit of those with severe mental illness on practice lists
Active participation in CPA

1.8.2 By not imposing limits on the number of out-patients attendances
By restricting their prescribing of recommended medication

1.8.3 Health of the Nation Mental Health Targets:
- to improve significantly the health and social functioning of mentally ill people
- to reduce the overall suicide rate by at least 15% by the year 2000
- to reduce the suicide rate of severely mentally ill people by at least 33% by the year 2000

Section 1.8: General Practitioner Fundholding

1.8.1   General practitioner fundholders (GPFHs) indicate their awareness of the needs   **A 0 1 2 3 4**
of those with severe mental illness and prioritise these needs

1.8.2   GPFHs ensure that patients with severe mental illness have access to high quality secondary services   **A 0 1 2 3 4**
and, wherever possible, involve themselves in the planning, monitoring and review of those services

1.8.3   GPFHs contribute to the attainment of Health of the Nation targets   **A 0 1 2 3 4**

SUMMARY RATING FOR SECTION 1.8:	**Scale B:**	**0**	**1**	**2**	**3**	**4**

Section 1.9 Assessment includes:

1.9.2   Statements in policy documents
Dedicated use of Mental Illness Specific Grant monies

1.9.3   e.g. through staff training

Section 1.9: Local Authority Social Services

1.9.1   Social Services Departments have a ring-fenced budget for purchasing mental   **A   0 1 2 3 4**
         health services

1.9.2   Social Services Departments agree the prioritisation of SMI   **A   0 1 2 3 4**

1.9.3   Social Services Departments endorse and actively support CPA and Care Management   **A   0 1 2 3 4**

SUMMARY RATING FOR SECTION 1.9:	**Scale B:**	**0**	**1**	**2**	**3**	**4**

Part 2: Providing Mental Health Services

2.1:   Community Services   0 1 2 3 4

2.2:   Rehabilitation & Activity   0 1 2 3 4

2.3:   Clinical Interventions   0 1 2 3 4

2.4:   Violence & Self-Harm   0 1 2 3 4

2.5:   Crisis Management   0 1 2 3 4

2.6:   Short-Stay Hospital Care   0 1 2 3 4

2.7:   Secure Longer Term Hospital Care   0 1 2 3 4

2.8:   Longer Term NHS (& NHS-Hostel) Accommodation   0 1 2 3 4

2.9:   Other (mostly non-NHS) Accommodation   0 1 2 3 4

2.10:	Clinical Records	0	1	2	3	4
2.11:	Local Health Service Audit Procedures	0	1	2	3	4
2.12:	Education of Mental Health Practitioners	0	1	2	3	4
2.13:	Local Community Issues	0	1	2	3	4
2.14:	Primary Care Liaison	0	1	2	3	4
2.15:	Social Services & other LA Departments	0	1	2	3	4
2.16:	Users, Carers & Voluntary Organisations	0	1	2	3	4
2.17:	Morale & Leadership	0	1	2	3	4

For rating scales please see fold out section at back of document

Section 2.1 Assessment includes:

2.1.1   Priority given to people with a diagnosis of schizophrenia or severe mental illness
Risk factors:
- serious violence
- serious self-harm
- serious self-neglect
- serious risk of exploitation
- specific relapse indicators

2.1.2   Management to:
- ensure priority
- formal written policy
- regular audit of caseload
- GPFH casemix

2.1.3   Written mental health assessment guidelines
Regular review (at least every 3 months)
Multidisciplinary review
Physical illness and disability assessed:
- general health
- poverty and/or self-neglect; diet, exercise, housing conditions, etc
- side-effects of medication
- regular (yearly) physical examination

2.1.4   Access available to both users and carers
Severely mentally ill have right of access to services - active list with telephone access, see Section 2.15

Section 2.1: Community Services

2.1.1   Access to community services is prioritised according to diagnosis and risk factors   **A   0   1   2   3   4**

2.1.2   Both clinical and fiscal management of caseload to allow time for the most disabled group   **A   0   1   2   3   4**

2.1.3   Regular multidisciplinary needs assessment is carried out for all at risk   **A   0   1   2   3   4**

2.1.4   There is a full range of legal, social, welfare and benefits advice and advocacy available to all   **A   0   1   2   3   4**
         service users

SUMMARY RATING FOR SECTION 2.1:	**Scale B:**	**0**	**1**	**2**	**3**	**4**

Section 2.2 Assessment includes:

2.2.1–5 Each offers good opportunities for treatment and rehabilitation

2.2.6 Activities other than 2.2.1-5 are provided specifically for people with severe mental illness

People with severe mental illness are actively encouraged to take part in these activities

Range of services provided:

- outings
- adult education
- lunch, social and drop in clubs
- training centres (e.g. basic numeracy and literacy classes)
- personal/domestic skills training
- voluntary work advocacy and befriending schemes

These services are effectively advertised

Local mental health workers are familiar with the range of services available

2.2.7 Range of weekend services provided

Transport provided

Services are effectively advertised

Both structured and unstructured

Special groups for women, young men, people from ethnic minorities etc.

Section 2.2: Rehabilitation & Activity

The following day care settings are available:

2.2.1   Day hospital   **H A / T / S S / V / P   A   0   1   2   3   4**

2.2.2   Day centre   **H A / T / S S / V / P   A   0   1   2   3   4**

2.2.3   Rehabilitation workshop   **H A / T / S S / V / P   A   0   1   2   3   4**

2.2.4   Sheltered workshop   **H A / T / S S / V / P   A   0   1   2   3   4**

2.2.5   Places in local industry   **H A / T / S S / V / P   A   0   1   2   3   4**

2.2.6   Opportunities for activities (both structured and unstructured) are made   **H A / T / S S / V / P   A   0   1   2   3   4**
        available to people with severe mental illness living in the community

2.2.7   Opportunities (as 2.2.6) are available during evenings and at weekends   **H A / T / S S / V / P   A   0   1   2   3   4**

SUMMARY RATING FOR SECTION 2.2:	**Scale B:**	0	1	2	3	4

Section 2.3 Assessment includes:

2.3.1   See British National Formulary sections 4.2.1 & 4.2.2
Budget for medication
Quality of depot clinic services

2.3.2   Clozapine, Respiradone
How many patients taking these drugs

2.3.3   People with severe mental illness have access to the full range of therapies:
- cognitive therapies
- behavioural therapies
- family interventions
- specialist psychosocial interventions for people with psychosis
- other techniques e.g. timeout, limited and maintained seclusion

Therapists are skilled and experienced in relevant methods
What proportion of current caseload have severe mental illness

2.3.4   See also Section 2.1

2.3.5   There are local prescribing guidelines
Sources of information regarding efficacy
Training of non-medical staff to recognise side-effects

Section 2.3: Clinical Interventions

2.3.1 A range of medication is available for the treatment of people with severe mental illness   **A   0 1 2 3 4**

2.3.2 A range of medication is available for those with treatment-resistant schizophrenia   **A   0 1 2 3 4**

2.3.3 A range of cognitive and behavioural therapies is available for people suffering from severe mental illness   **A   0 1 2 3 4**

2.3.4 Medication is routinely assessed as part of regular multidisciplinary team review   **A   0 1 2 3 4**

2.3.5 Review of medication includes efficacy and side-effects   **A   0 1 2 3 4**

SUMMARY RATING FOR SECTION 2.3:	Scale B:	0	1	2	3	4

Section 2.4 Assessment includes:

2.4.1   Examples

Must be accessible to all those who need to know

2.4.2   Follow up includes action recorded in case notes

Examples seen

2.4.3   See also Section 2.11

2.4.4   Anticipation, prevention and diffusion techniques

Control and restraint techniques

Staff are debriefed following violent incidents

Support to staff following violent incidents

2.4.5   Adequate staffing levels

Adequate security

Rapid isolation

Unhindered observation

Alarm systems

2.4.6   All clinical staff are trained

Training for medical staff other than as part of basic training

Staff are debriefed following incidents of suicide

Support to staff following incidents of suicide

Section 2.4: Violence & Self-Harm

2.4.1   Violent incidents are recorded in confidential records other than patient notes but readily accessible when needed   **A 0 1 2 3 4**

2.4.2   Incidents reported by carers are logged and followed-up   **A 0 1 2 3 4**

2.4.3   All incidents of suicide, serious self-harm and violence are subject to regular audit review   **A 0 1 2 3 4**

2.4.4   Staff in mental health teams are trained in the management of violent situations   **A 0 1 2 3 4**

2.4.5   Units at particular risk of violence or self-harm are appropriately designed   **A 0 1 2 3 4**

2.4.6   All clinical staff are trained in the management of suicidal patients and serious self-harm   **A 0 1 2 3 4**

SUMMARY RATING FOR SECTION 2.4:	**Scale B:**	0	1	2	3	4

Section 2.5 Assessment includes:

2.5.1   Separate area for assessment

Specifically trained staff

Specifically designed room and furnishings

Provides 24 hour local cover

2.5.2   Inspect the place of safety

How often is it used ?

Separate area for assessment

Specifically trained staff

Specifically designed room and furnishings

2.5.3   Formal arrangement/outreach service

Variation in cover between different CMHTs

Multidisciplinary approach

How is service contacted

Who responds – appropriate numbers of people, with appropriate skill mix

Section 2.5: Crisis Management

2.5.1   There is appropriate accommodation for the assessment of people in psychiatric crisis   **A   0   1   2   3   4**

2.5.2   The designated place of safety (S.136) is appropriate for assessing people in crisis   **A   0   1   2   3   4**

2.5.3   Skilled staff can respond 24 hours a day for assessing people in psychiatric crisis in domiciliary or other settings   **A   0   1   2   3   4**

2.5.4   Approved social workers are readily available for Mental Health Act assessments   **C   0   1   2   3   4   5   6   7**

2.5.5   Section 12 approved doctors are readily available for Mental Health Act assessments   **C   0   1   2   3   4   5   6   7**

SUMMARY RATING FOR SECTION 2.5:	**Scale B:**	0	1	2	3	4

35

Section 2.6: Short-Stay Hospital Care

Local sites _____ PAG _____ C 0 1 2 3 4 5 6 7

_____ PAG _____ C 0 1 2 3 4 5 6 7

_____ PAG _____ C 0 1 2 3 4 5 6 7

_____ PAG _____ C 0 1 2 3 4 5 6 7

Separate secure accommodation for 'intensive care' is available for those whose behaviour C 0 1 2 3 4 5 6 7
is temporarily threatening, self-harming, severely overactive or sexually harassing

A 0 1 2 3 4

SUMMARY RATING FOR SECTION 2.6:	Scale B:	0	1	2	3	4

Section 2.7: Secure Longer Term Hospital Care

Local sites _____ PAG _____ **C 0 1 2 3 4 5 6 7**

_____ PAG _____ **C 0 1 2 3 4 5 6 7**

_____ PAG _____ **C 0 1 2 3 4 5 6 7**

_____ PAG _____ **C 0 1 2 3 4 5 6 7**

Accommodation is available for people who pose a serious risk of danger to others and/or require   **C 0 1 2 3 4 5 6 7**
intensive care for a longer period than would be appropriate for an intensive care ward

         A 0 1 2 3 4

SUMMARY RATING FOR SECTION 2.7:	Scale B:	0	1	2	3	4

Section 2.8: Longer-Stay NHS (& NHS-Hostel) Accommodation

Local sites _____ PAG _____ C 0 1 2 3 4 5 6 7

_____ PAG _____ C 0 1 2 3 4 5 6 7

_____ PAG _____ C 0 1 2 3 4 5 6 7

_____ PAG _____ C 0 1 2 3 4 5 6 7

Residential places are available for people whose behaviour or poor living skills mean that   C 0 1 2 3 4 5 6 7
they need constant supervision; in particular from trained nursing staff awake at night

A 0 1 2 3 4

SUMMARY RATING FOR SECTION 2.8:	Scale B:	0	1	2	3	4

Section 2.9: Other (mostly non-NHS) Accommodation

2.9.1   Short-stay accommodation (< 6 months) with sleep-in and day staff   **C 0 1 2 3 4 5 6 7**

_____ PAG _____ **HA / T / SS / V / P**

_____ PAG _____ **HA / T / SS / V / P**

_____ PAG _____ **HA / T / SS / V / P**

2.9.2:   Long-stay (> 6 months) accommodation with sleep-in and day staff   **C 0 1 2 3 4 5 6 7**

_____ PAG _____ **HA / T / SS / V / P**

_____ PAG _____ **HA / T / SS / V / P**

_____ PAG _____ **HA / T / SS / V / P**

continued

2.9.3: Day staffed residential hostel   **C   0 1 2 3 4 5 6 7**

_____ PAG _____   **H A / T / S S / V / P**

_____ PAG _____   **H A / T / S S / V / P**

_____ PAG _____   **H A / T / S S / V / P**

2.9.4: Group homes or similar with up to daily visiting   **C   0 1 2 3 4 5 6 7**

_____ PAG _____   **H A / T / S S / V / P**

_____ PAG _____   **H A / T / S S / V / P**

_____ PAG _____   **H A / T / S S / V / P**

continued

2.9.5:   Group homes or similar with on-call facilities only   **C   0 1 2 3 4 5 6 7**

_____ PAG _____   **HA / T / SS / V / P**

_____ PAG _____   **HA / T / SS / V / P**

_____ PAG _____   **HA / T / SS / V / P**

2.9.6:   Bedsits or lodgings with supervised standards for use by people with severe mental illness   **C   0 1 2 3 4 5 6 7**

_____ PAG _____   **HA / T / SS / V / P**

_____ PAG _____   **HA / T / SS / V / P**

_____ PAG _____   **HA / T / SS / V / P**

SUMMARY RATING FOR SECTION 2.9:	**Scale B:**	**0**	**1**	**2**	**3**	**4**

Section 2.10 Assessment includes:

2.10.1 0 - Little or no evidence of systematic recording for service support

1 - Active steps being taken but not so far implemented

2 - Some specific functions supported and partially integrated between teams/settings

3 - The CPA is fully supported and integrated

4 - A fully supported and integrated district MHIS

2.10.2 Service functions: CPA, supervision registers, Mental Health Act, supervised discharge (when appropriate), referral letters, problem lists, care plans, discharge summaries, planning, patient centred interrogation, audit, statistics, information transfer

2.10.3 Consider both computerised and paper based systems

Data Protection Act

Secretarial notes, word processing systems and mail

Removal and transport of notes from main site

2.10.4 Location of medical records: staff office; central office

Access to records: formal/informal request; shared systems

2.10.5 See also Sections 2.1, 2.14 & 2.15

Section 2.10: Clinical Records

2.10.1 Rate degree of implementation of mental health information systems for service use. **0 1 2 3 4**

(See notes for rating scale)

2.10.2 The district has a specialist mental health record system that effectively supports basic clinical and service functions. **A   0 1 2 3 4**

2.10.3 There are adequate precautions in place to maintain the security and confidentiality of all patient information. **A   0 1 2 3 4**

2.10.4 All authorised staff have ready access to patient records. **A   0 1 2 3 4**

2.10.5 There are links for information transfer between: **A   0 1 2 3 4**
- social services and health services
- hospital and community providers
- primary and secondary care

2.10.6 The Data Protection Act is fully observed and patients and relatives have access to medical records **A   0 1 2 3 4**

SUMMARY RATING FOR SECTION 2.10:	Scale B:	0	1	2	3	4

Section 2.11 Assessment includes:

2.11.3 Examine the criteria
e.g. see Section 2.11.4

2.11.4 e.g. Discharge planning to meet the requirements of CPA & Mental Health Act
Service co-ordination to ensure that care plans derived from assessment of need are fulfilled
Systematic audits to monitor the quality of routine clinical care
Audit of adverse events
Monitoring of relevant local statistics

2.11.5 Consider both medical and clinical audit

Section 2.11: Local Health Service Audit Procedures

2.11.1 There is a written programme of audit activities for the year   **A 0 1 2 3 4**

2.11.2 There is a functioning audit committee that meets regularly with a stated agenda and   **A 0 1 2 3 4**
clear links with all professions and the Chief Executive of the Trust

2.11.3 There are clear criteria for selecting audit topics   **A 0 1 2 3 4**

2.11.4 Audit activities over the past 12 months have included services for the severely mentally ill   **A 0 1 2 3 4**

2.11.5 The audit programme includes a majority of multidisciplinary projects   **A 0 1 2 3 4**

SUMMARY RATING FOR SECTION 2.11:	**Scale B:**	**0**	**1**	**2**	**3**	**4**

45

Section 2.12 Assessment includes:

2.12.1 The educational plan is regularly updated

Educational opportunities are audited

2.12.2 Postgraduate medical education facilities

Opportunities to attend external courses and conferences

Training for professional qualifications e.g. Royal College membership

Links with academic institutions

Record of published research

2.12.3 Training to manage violent and potentially violent situations

Training in the management of self-harm

Refresher courses

Exchanges between agencies and/or settings

Opportunities to attend external courses and conferences

Links with academic institutions

Training for professional qualifications

2.12.4 Basic knowledge of psychopharmacology

Training in risk assessment

Ability to recognise prodromal symptoms

Training in basic family interventions

Is training a basic requirement for becoming a keyworker?

2.12.5 User and carer organisations asked to provide presentations or to assist in running workshops.

Section 2.12: Education of Mental Health Practitioners

2.12.1 For all professions, there is a plan or policy, and an identifiable budget, for education and professional development   **A 0 1 2 3 4**

2.12.2 A range of educational opportunities exists for all medical staff, appropriate to their professional development   **A 0 1 2 3 4**

2.12.3 A range of educational opportunities exists for all non-medical staff, appropriate to their needs and professional development   **A 0 1 2 3 4**

2.12.4 All local keyworkers have received basic training appropriate to their role   **A 0 1 2 3 4**

2.12.5 Local users and carers are involved in the training of mental health professionals   **A 0 1 2 3 4**

SUMMARY RATING FOR SECTION 2.12:	**Scale B:**	0	1	2	3	4

Section 2.13 Assessment includes:

2.13.1   Extent of local homeless problem (If very low, rate 9)
  Permanence of projects/long term support
  Availability of flexible/suitable housing
  Jointly funded projects (e.g. Health & Social Services or voluntary)

2.13.2   Advocacy/befriending schemes
  Permanence of projects
  Vetting of project participants
  Support from voluntary organisations

2.13.3   Written information for users and carers in relevant language(s) about:
  • Mental Health Act
  • illness (symptoms, prognosis etc,)
  • medication (dosage, side effects, administration)
  • services

2.13.4   Interpreters are competent. Non-clinical hospital staff, professional interpreters
  Interpreters are trained to help with interviews with the severely mentally ill
  Interpreters are properly supported and debriefed
  Interpreting services can respond quickly if needed
  Appropriateness and cost of interpreting service

2.13.5   Knowledge of local non-medical services
  Knowledge of local epidemiology (unemployment, ethnic minorities, housing, poverty, isolation etc.)
  Knowledge of specific issues relating to mental illness (diagnosis, treatment etc.)

Section 2.13: Local Community Issues

2.13.1 Appropriate care is directed specifically at homeless and roofless people suffering from severe mental illness

A   0   1   2   3   4

HA / T / SS / P / V

2.13.2 There is a deliberate effort to contact people in the community suffering from severe mental illness but not in touch with services.

A   0   1   2   3   4

HA / T / SS / P / V

2.13.3 A full range of translated information exists for patients from ethnic minorities

A   0   1   2   3   4

2.13.4 Trained and supported interpreters are readily available to help deal with patients who do not speak English

A   0   1   2   3   4

2.13.5 Mental health professionals are knowledgeable about local community issues and epidemiology

A   0   1   2   3   4

SUMMARY RATING FOR SECTION 2.13:	Scale B:	0	1	2	3	4

Section 2.14 Assessment includes:

2.14.1 Service directories
Other communications – newsletters etc.
Regular meetings with representative of CMHT
CPNs based in primary care

2.14.3 GP registers of people with severe mental illness
Quality of links between primary and secondary care
Agreed procedure
Audit of referrals and caseloads (see 2.1.2)

Section 2.14: Primary Care Liaison

2.14.1   There is effective communication between primary and secondary care teams   **A   0 1 2 3 4**

2.14.2   Joint primary-secondary audit activities are carried out   **A   0 1 2 3 4**

2.14.3   There are priority arrangements for referring patients with severe mental illness   **A   0 1 2 3 4**

SUMMARY RATING FOR SECTION 2.14:	Scale B:	0	1	2	3	4

Section 2.15 Assessment includes:

2.15.1 Social workers are trained to use the following schemes:
- CPA (enough trained keyworkers)
- Mental Health Act (ASWs)
- Care Management

2.15.2 See example of practice protocols

2.15.3 CMHTs with full or part-time social worker

2.15.4 Examples of effective inter-agency working:
- joint care planning
- active involvement in shared care
- joint information collection
- joint information systems
- joint commissioning

Section 2.15: Social Services & other LA Departments

2.15.1   Enough local social workers are trained to help the severely mentally ill   **A   0 1 2 3 4**

2.15.2   Clear practice protocols exist for dealing with severe mental illness   **A   0 1 2 3 4**

2.15.3   Social workers play an active role within local CMHTs   **A   0 1 2 3 4**

2.15.4   There is effective inter-agency working between local health and social services   **A   0 1 2 3 4**

SUMMARY RATING FOR SECTION 2.15:	**Scale B:**	**0**	**1**	**2**	**3**	**4**

Section 2.16 Assessment includes:

2.16.1   Provision of office space
Use of meeting rooms
Accommodation for day activities
Providing clinical staff with time to give talks, workshops etc.

2.16.2   Contacts with both individuals and organisations
Training of users and carers to assist with committee work
Participation in planning services/quality assurance and audit
Formal mechanisms for feedback on comments

2.16.3   Aimed at individuals and organisation/groups
Access to mental health professionals for information and advice
Information/education about illness
Information/education about medication and side-effects
Information about Mental Health Act (poster presentations on wards not sufficient)
Information and advice about local services (NHS and Non-NHS)
Information about welfare, benefits, lodgings etc.

2.16.4   As for 2.16.3

2.16.5   Route for referral to respite care
Appropriateness of accommodation

2.16.6   Access to therapeutic services e.g. counselling, family therapy
Outreach. Advocacy. Support groups & meetings
Provision of Crisis Cards
Education - recognising relapse, prodromal symptoms, side-effects of medication

Section 2.16: Users, Carers & Voluntary Organisations

2.16.1   Local voluntary organisations are assisted to provide services for the severely mentally ill   **A   0   1   2   3   4**

HA / T / SS / V / P

2.16.2   Local users, carers and voluntary organisations actively participate in Trust affairs   **A   0   1   2   3   4**

2.16.3   Patients/clients have information and education appropriate to their needs   **A   0   1   2   3   4**

2.16.4   Carers have information and education appropriate to their needs, both about their relatives/friends and in general   **A   0   1   2   3   4**

2.16.5   An appropriate range of respite facilities allows users and/or carers a planned period away from stressful or tiring situations   **A   0   1   2   3   4**

2.16.6   Support is offered to carers   **A   0   1   2   3   4**

SUMMARY RATING FOR SECTION 2.16:	**Scale B:**	**0**	**1**	**2**	**3**	**4**

Section 2.17 Assessment includes:

2.17.2   Managers are approachable and available to staff

Managers and staff share ownership in the vision, understand and approve it

2.17.3   Levels of uncertified sick leave

Manager and staff turnover - length in post

Use of locums

2.17.4   Responsibility for budgets is allocated to the person with responsibility for the relevant action

2.17.6   Clinical staff are involved from early stages, more than just information or consultation

They have direct access to representatives from the purchasing organisation

2.17.7   Satisfactory procedures for face to face discussions, minuted if necessary, to resolve problems

Staff agree that morale is high, even if there are problems e.g. of resources, etc.

2.17.9   Working 'to the book' is not taken literally. There is room for innovation and for personal initiative

Section 2.17: Morale & Leadership

2.17.1 There is shared vision between executives of purchasing and providing bodies   **A 0 1 2 3 4**

2.17.2 There is commitment to clear aims and achievable targets with an open style of management   **A 0 1 2 3 4**

2.17.3 There is organisational stability   **A 0 1 2 3 4**

2.17.4 True budgeting control is devolved down to the most appropriate level   **A 0 1 2 3 4**

2.17.5 There is strong clinical leadership in all professions   **A 0 1 2 3 4**

2.17.6 Clinical staff are involved in contracting and decision making   **A 0 1 2 3 4**

2.17.7 Clinical staff have reasonable control of their job   **A 0 1 2 3 4**

2.17.8 Resources are adequate to achieve good standards of care   **A 0 1 2 3 4**

2.17.9 There are opportunities to develop new projects and ideas   **A 0 1 2 3 4**

SUMMARY RATING FOR SECTION 2.17:	Scale B:	0	1	2	3	4

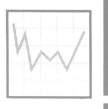

GLOSSARY

A&C: Administrative and Clerical

A&E: Accident & Emergency

ASW: Approved Social Worker

C&R: Control & Restraint

CMHN: Community Mental Health Nurse

CMHT: Community Mental Health Team

CPA: Care Programme Approach

CPN: Community Psychiatric Nurse

CRU: College Research Unit

CSAG: Clinical Standards Advisory Group

CSAG-S: Clinical Standards Advisory Group – Schizophrenia Study

DGH: District General Hospital

DHA: District Health Authority

DMU: NHS Directly Managed Unit

ECR: Extra Contractual Referral

FCE: Finished Consultant Episodes

FHSA: Family Health Services Authority

GP: General Practitioner

GPFH: General Practice Fund Holder

HAS: Health Advisory Service

HIP: Health Investment Plan

IT: Information Technology

LASS: Local Authority Social Services

MDO: Mentally Disordered Offender

MDT: Multidisciplinary Team

MHA: Mental Health Act (1983)

MHAC: Mental Health Act Commission

MHS: Mental Health Service

MIAG: Mental Illness Action Group

OT: Occupational Therapy

PAS: Patient Administration System

RCPsych: Royal College of Psychiatrists

RSU: Regional Secure Unit

S117 MHA: Section 117 of the Mental Health Act (1983)

S133 MHA: Section 133 of the Mental Health Act (1983)

S136 MHA: Section 136 of the Mental Health Act (1983)

UPA8: Underprivileged Areas Score (Jarman indices)

SCZ: Schizophrenia

SMI: Severe Mental Illness

SSD: Social Service Department

SW: Social Work

Advocacy - the comunicating of expressed needs by, or on behalf of, a user to service providers.

Audit - "The systematic critical analysis of the quality of care, including the procedures used for diagnosis and treatment, the use of resources, and the resulting outcome and quality of life for the patient" (DOH 1989)

Carer - a relative or friend of a user who is actively involved in their care.

Care Management - from the 1st April 1993 local authority social service departments have become the lead agency responsible for assessing, purchasing and monitoring the community care of people with disabilities linked to mental illness, old age, physical disabilities and learning difficulties. Social Service Inspectorate guidelines identify seven core tasks of care management: publishing information; determining the level of assessment needed; assessing need; care planning; implementing the care plan; monitoring and review. There is considerable flexibility in the way each authority can structure care management. However, authorities are expected to produce community care plans consistent with those of health authorities, and to produce individual care packages in collaboration with medical, nursing and other relevant groups.

Case Management - similar to care management; assessment and care planning is carried out by a case manager who co-ordinates the delivery of care and is responsible for monitoring and review. A case manager may also act as a key worker.

Clozapine - a recently introduced psychotropic drug still under test currently used to treat treatment-resistant schizophrenia.

Community Mental Health Nurse - see Community Psychiatric Nurse.

CPA: Care Programme Approach - the Care Programme Approach was introduced in the NHS in April 1991. Health Care Providers are required to develop, in collaboration with local social services departments, individual packages of care (care programmes) for all in-patients about to be discharged from hospital and all new patients accepted by the specialist psychiatric services. Care programmes may range from 'minimal' single worker assessment and monitoring, for individuals with less severe mental health and social needs, to complex multidisciplinary assessments and treatment.

CRU: College Research Unit - an independent multidisciplinary research unit attached to the Royal College of Psychiatrists. Commissioned to draft standards and provide research and office support for the CSAG schizophrenia study.

CSAG: Clinical Standards Advisory Group – The CSAG was established in 1991 under S62 of the NHS and Community Care Act as an independent source of expert advice to UK Health Ministers and NHS bodies on standards of clinical care for, and on access and availability of services to, NHS patients. The remit to study services for people with schizophrenia (CSAG-S) was set in August 1993.

DMU: Directly Managed Unit (NHS) – A hospital or community provider service which has not yet sought or achieved Trust status. DMUs remain under the management of DHAs, although in other respects, the "purchaser-provider" separation is identical to Trusts.

FCE: Finished Consultant Episodes – The point at which a patient is referred back to the care of a GP or other specialist service and a discharge report completed.

GPFH: General Practice Fund Holder – GP practices with lists above a certain size are free to apply for their own NHS budget to obtain a defined range of services. Budgets also cover practice staff costs, improvement to premises and drug costs.

Keyworker – An identified person who has a defined responsibility towards a specific user of services, usually with some responsibility for service provision and monitoring of care.

Outreach – services which rely primarily on home visiting and in vivo interventions.

Perverse Incentives – contractual agreements which may encourage service providers to adopt practices or policies that run counter to good clinical management e.g. extra funding for increased length of in-patient stay, the use of episode based monitoring (FCEs) as a contract currency.

S117 MHA: Section 117 of the Mental Health Act 1983 – Section 117 applies to individuals detained under Section 3, 37, 47 or 48 who cease to be detained and are discharged from hospital. It is the responsibility of the RMO to ensure a keyworker is nominated and provides after-care services, in conjunction with local authority social services, until they are satisfied that the individual no longer needs such care.

S133 MHA: Section 133 of the Mental Health Act 1983 – Section 133 places a duty on managers of hospitals to inform nearest relatives of the discharge of detained patients where practicable, unless the patient or relative has requested otherwise.

S136 MHA: Section 136 of the Mental Health Act 1983 – a police officer can detain a person in a public place who appears to be "suffering from mental disorder" and is in "immediate need of care or control", and remove them to "a place of safety".

UPA8: Underprivileged Areas Score (Jarman indices) - The UPA8 is based on eight census indices, being the percentage of people in the local population with the following characteristics: people aged 65+; children aged <4; social class 5; unemployed; single-parent households; overcrowding; highly mobile people; and ethnic minorities. Each item is weighted according to GP's views of how much they think it contributes to their workload. The weighted sum, standardised and normalised, constitutes the "Jarman score". The score can be used as an indicator of deprivation in a geographically defined population and as an approximate indicator of morbidity.

Special Hospital - hospitals for psychiatric patients who require care in conditions of special security. In England, 3 hospitals are managed by the Special Hospitals Services Authority: Broadmoor; Rampton; and Ashworth. In Scotland there is a State Hospital at Carstairs.

Supervision Register - from April 1st 1994 all Purchasers and Providers of Mental Health Services are required to have in place a register which ensures the identification and registration of all severely mentally ill people at risk of causing serious harm to themselves or others or of serious neglect.

User - a person with a mental health problem who is receiving mental health care services.

Scale A: Action to meet guideline

0	No action yet taken, few plans
1	Plans, little action
2	Guideline is partially met
3	Guideline is substantially met
4	Guideline is fully met or exceeded
9	Not known or not applicable

Scale B: Overall quality of service

0	Unacceptable
1	Poor
2	Fair
3	Good
4	Excellent
9	Not known or not applicable

Scale C: If an authorised care worker requested the specified service today, how long would a patient or client wait before it became available?

0	No such service available
1	1 year+
2	3-12 months
3	1-3 months
4	1-4 weeks
5	1-7 days
6	<24 hours
7	<1 hour
9	Not known or not applicable

Scale D: Who is providing the service?

HA	Health authority/other health purchaser
T	Trust/hospital/other NHS provider
SS	Social services/local authority
V	Voluntary organisation
P	Private sector

PAG Scale: Quality of residential accommodation

Rate each item

0	Poor
1	Adequate
2	Good
9	Not applicable

— Information about telephone helplines
— Accommodation is domestic in style
— A variety of daytime activities is available
— Access to private outdoor space
— Private single-sex bathing facilities
— Private single-sex toilet facilities
— Appropriate staffing ratios
— Appropriate staffing skill mix
— Staff seen active on the ward
— Enough single rooms
— Comfortable and good decor
— Fosters independence
— Quality/quantity staff/patient interaction
— Personalised care
— Consultation with users
— Flexible routines
— Adequate time off wards
— Information on MHA, benefits, welfare
— Buildings designed appropriately
— Quality of food
— Access to smoking/non-smoking areas
— Adequate levels of safety and security
— Access to therapies
— Quiet room
— Space to meet privately with visitors
— Private access to telephone

Printed in the United Kingdom for HMSO

Dd 0301186   C280   8/95   65536   328989   28/33218